MEDITERRANEAN DIET FOR HEALTHY LIVING

Unlock Vibrant Living Through Proven Recipes, Nutritional Insights, And Lifestyle Tips - Your Key To Longevity And Wellness

JEMMA KEIRA

CONTENTS

CHAPTER ONE 8

Introduction 8

Advantages Of The Mediterranean Diet 8

Key Mediterranean Diet Principles 10

The Mediterranean Diet For Longevity 13

CHAPTER TWO...16

Wine Moderation: A Salute To Heart Health..16

Limiting Red Meat: Protein Balance For Longevity...17

Dairy In Moderation: A Healthy Approach To Calcium Consumption....................................18

Herbs And Spices From The Mediterranean: Flavorful Medicine For The Body 20

CHAPTER THREE 22

The Emphasis On Appropriate Hydration For Healthy Living On The Mediterranean Diet 22

The Mediterranean Diet's Social And Lifestyle Aspects For Healthy Living 24

Weight Control 26

Precautions And Potential Health Risks 28

CHAPTER FOUR...30

A Mediterranean Diet For Every Stage Of Life 30

Including The Mediterranean Diet In Your Daily Life 31

Meal Plans For The Mediterranean Diet 33

Mediterranean Diet-Inspired Recipes 34

THE END 39

DISCLAIMER

The information provided in this book is for general informational purposes only and is not intended as a substitute for professional medical advice or treatment. It is important to consult with a qualified healthcare professional before making any dietary or lifestyle changes, especially if you have any underlying health conditions or concerns.

The author and publisher of this book are not responsible for any adverse effects or consequences resulting from the use of the information presented herein. The information in this book is based on the author's personal experiences and research, and it is important to understand that individual results may vary.

Any references to specific brands, products, or websites are only made for illustrative purposes only and do not constitute endorsements. The reader is encouraged to conduct independent research and make informed decisions.

The content of this book is meant to provide guidance and suggestions related to vegan diets, nutrition, and health. Readers are encouraged to use their discretion and consult with a healthcare professional or registered dietitian for personalized advice and recommendations. The author and publisher make no warranties, expressed or implied, regarding the accuracy or completeness of the information presented in this book and disclaim any liability for any loss, injury, or damage incurred as a consequence of using the information provided.

By reading this book, you acknowledge and agree to the terms of this disclaimer. It is your responsibility to make informed decisions about your health and dietary choices, and you should seek professional guidance when needed.

CHAPTER ONE

Introduction

The Mediterranean diet is more than simply a culinary trend; it's a way of life that has been linked to a slew of health advantages. This diet, which originated in the traditional dietary patterns of Mediterranean Sea-bordering nations such as Greece, Italy, and Spain, has garnered global attention for its ability to boost general well-being. The Mediterranean diet, distinguished by an abundance of fresh fruits and vegetables, whole grains, healthy fats, and lean meats, stands out as a tasty and sustainable method to promote a healthy lifestyle.

Advantages Of The Mediterranean Diet

The Mediterranean diet is well-known for its beneficial effects on several facets of health. One of its significant advantages is its ability to support heart health. This diet has regularly been demonstrated in studies to minimize the risk of heart disease by lowering LDL (bad) cholesterol levels and blood pressure. The concentration of heart-healthy fats found in olive oil and almonds contributes to these beneficial benefits.

In addition, the Mediterranean diet is linked to a decreased risk of chronic illnesses such as type 2 diabetes. A diet high in fiber-rich foods, such as fruits, vegetables, and whole grains, aids with blood sugar regulation and insulin sensitivity. This not only helps with diabetes prevention but also helps with weight control, which is an important element of overall health.

Another area where the Mediterranean diet excels is cognitive performance. The combination of omega-3 fatty acids from fish and antioxidants from fruits and vegetables has been associated with a lower risk of cognitive decline and neurodegenerative disorders like Alzheimer's.

The Mediterranean diet has been linked to better mental well-being in addition to physical health. Consuming nutrient-dense foods, as well as the social component of sharing meals with family and friends, helps to maintain a happy mental attitude. Furthermore, the diet's ability to lower inflammation in the body may help with mental wellness.

Key Mediterranean Diet Principles

The Mediterranean diet is a flexible framework that promotes particular food groups and lifestyle choices rather than a rigorous set of guidelines. Understanding its fundamental concepts is critical for properly implementing this approach to healthy living.

1. Plant-based foods are emphasized:

The Mediterranean diet is centered on plant-based foods as its foundation. Fruits and vegetables take the spotlight, delivering a plethora of vitamins, minerals, and antioxidants. These foods not only improve general health, but they also provide brilliant colors and tastes to meals. Whole grains, legumes, nuts, and seeds supplement the plant-based focus by providing a range of minerals and fiber.

2. Fats that are good for you:

Healthy fats, particularly those found in olive oil, almonds, and fatty fish, are emphasized in the Mediterranean diet. Olive oil, a mainstay in this diet, is high in monounsaturated fats, which have been linked to heart health.

Incorporating modest amounts of nuts and seeds adds beneficial fats, while fatty fish like salmon and mackerel supply omega-3 fatty acids, which are vital for heart and brain function.

3. Proteins that are low in fat:

The Mediterranean diet's protein sources are lean and diversified. Red and processed meats are favored above fish and shellfish, poultry, lentils, and nuts. Because of its omega-3 concentration, fish, in particular, is an important component. This protein balance promotes muscular health while lowering the intake of saturated fats present in red meat.

4. Grain Whole:

Whole grains are an important part of the Mediterranean diet because they provide a consistent supply of energy and key elements. Refined grains are chosen over whole wheat bread, brown rice, quinoa, and bulgur. Whole grains provide improved digestion, consistent energy levels, and a decreased risk of chronic illnesses.

Finally, the Mediterranean diet provides a comprehensive approach to healthy living by combining delicious and varied meals with significant health advantages. Individuals may improve their physical well-being while also enjoying a sustainable and culturally rich way of eating by prioritizing plant-based foods, healthy fats, lean meats, and whole grains. Adopting the Mediterranean diet's core principles may be a tasty path toward a healthier, more vibrant existence.

The Mediterranean Diet For Longevity

The Mediterranean diet is well-known for its multiple health advantages, which promote not just physical well-being but also total lifespan. This dietary pattern, inspired by the traditional eating patterns of communities living along the Mediterranean Sea, includes a wide range of foods that contribute to a healthy and balanced lifestyle. In this examination, we will look at various components of the Mediterranean diet and how they contribute to the general health and well-being of people who follow this way of life.

Fruits and vegetables: The Foundations of Mediterranean Diet

Fruits and vegetables are at the core of the Mediterranean diet, acting as the principal sources of important vitamins, minerals, and antioxidants. This diet's abundance of fresh produce gives a wide range of health advantages, including enhanced cardiovascular health, a stronger immune system, and a lower risk of chronic illnesses.

The bright hues of Mediterranean fruits and vegetables indicate the presence of phytochemicals, which are anti-inflammatory and disease-fighting agents.

The Mediterranean diet promotes the eating of a wide variety of fruits and vegetables, with a focus on seasonal and locally available foods. This not only benefits local agriculture but also guarantees that people get a range of nutrients all year.

Incorporating a colorful variety of vegetables such as tomatoes, peppers, leafy greens, and fruits such as citrus, berries, and figs into meals adds taste as well as nutritional richness, making the Mediterranean diet a tasty and beneficial choice.

CHAPTER TWO

Wine Moderation: A Salute To Heart Health

The modest use of red wine, which is commonly savored during meals, is one of the Mediterranean diet's distinguishing features. Red wine has been linked to a variety of health advantages, especially when drank in moderation. It includes polyphenols, such as resveratrol, which are known to have antioxidant and anti-inflammatory effects. These substances promote healthy blood vessels and lower the risk of heart disease, which benefits cardiovascular health.

Moderation is the key to getting the advantages of wine in the Mediterranean diet. Excessive alcohol consumption can be harmful to one's health, thus it's important to follow established guidelines. A modest consumption, usually one glass per day for women and up to two glasses per day for men, may be part of a healthy lifestyle, bringing a touch of conviviality to meals while boosting heart health.

Limiting Red Meat: Protein Balance For Longevity

The Mediterranean diet limits red meat intake in favor of leaner protein sources such as fish, poultry, lentils, and nuts. Red and processed meat consumption has been linked to a decreased risk of chronic illnesses such as cardiovascular disease and some forms of cancer. Fish, which is high in omega-3 fatty acids, is a cornerstone of the Mediterranean diet and helps with brain health, inflammation reduction, and general well-being.

Individuals can maintain a balanced intake of key nutrients without the possible downsides associated with excessive red meat consumption by prioritizing plant-based proteins and including fish in their diet. This nutritional strategy not only promotes personal health but also corresponds with ecologically friendly and sustainable methods.

Dairy In Moderation: A Healthy Approach To Calcium Consumption

While dairy products are part of the Mediterranean diet, they are consumed in moderation. The emphasis is on high-quality dairy products like Greek yogurt and cheese, which give important minerals like calcium and protein. These dairy options are frequently fermented, which promotes intestinal health by containing helpful bacteria.

The Mediterranean diet encourages moderate dairy consumption since, while dairy may be a significant source of nutrients, overconsumption may lead to certain health problems. Individuals may enjoy the advantages of dairy without compromising overall health by selecting high-quality, nutrient-dense dairy alternatives and including them in a well-rounded diet.

Fresh and local foods are important for nourishing both the body and the community.

The emphasis on fresh, locally sourced foods is a core tenet of the Mediterranean diet. This not only guarantees that nutrient-dense and seasonal produce is consumed, but it also benefits local farmers and communities.

Individuals contribute to sustainable agriculture, lessen their environmental effects, and enjoy the freshest and most tasty foods by purchasing locally farmed fruits, vegetables, and other food items.

The Mediterranean diet promotes a connection between people and their food, cultivating an appreciation for the origin and quality of each element.

This mindful eating strategy fosters a greater knowledge of food's influence on health and the environment, making it a comprehensive and sustainable lifestyle option.

Herbs And Spices From The Mediterranean: Flavorful Medicine For The Body

Herbs and spices play an important part in the Mediterranean diet, not just for flavor but also for adding to the diet's overall health advantages. Herbs like basil, oregano, rosemary, and thyme, as well as spices like garlic and cinnamon, lend richness to recipes while also supplying antioxidants and anti-inflammatory components.

Many Mediterranean herbs and spices have been linked to a variety of health advantages, including better digestion, immunological support, and illness prevention. The inclusion of these savory ingredients in meals not only improves the gastronomic experience but also benefits the general well-being of people who follow the Mediterranean diet.

Finally, the Mediterranean diet is more than a culinary legacy; it is a way of life that promotes health, longevity, and sustainability. The Mediterranean diet, with its variety of fruits and vegetables and moderate use of wine, provides a comprehensive approach to nutrition that can be both fun and nourishing. Individuals may engage on a path toward greater health by adopting these dietary guidelines, relishing the rich flavors and many advantages of this time-tested method of eating.

CHAPTER THREE

The Emphasis On Appropriate Hydration For Healthy Living On The Mediterranean Diet

The emphasis on appropriate hydration is an often neglected but critical part of the Mediterranean diet. While the diet focuses mostly on nutritious meals, the necessity of staying hydrated cannot be emphasized. The Mediterranean region's warm temperature emphasizes the importance of a well-balanced fluid intake for general health and well-being.

Water is a popular beverage in Mediterranean civilizations. It is an essential component of a healthy lifestyle and supplements the diet's nutrient-rich meals. Water is essential for several physiological activities, such as digestion, nutrition absorption, and temperature control. Staying hydrated also benefits cardiovascular health, renal function, and cognitive ability.

Herbal teas, in addition to water, are widely taken in the Mediterranean diet, offering not just hydration but also possible health advantages. Chamomile and mint teas, for example, are well-known in the region for their relaxing and digestive effects. These beverages not only help with hydration consumption, but they also provide a tasty and culturally rich element to everyday life.

Individuals are advised to listen to their bodies and drink when thirsty with the Mediterranean diet to guarantee appropriate hydration. This intuitive approach is consistent with the diet's broader philosophy, which stresses mindful eating and listening to the body's natural indications. While water is the most common beverage, moderate drinking of red wine, a cornerstone of the Mediterranean diet, can also help to increase total fluid intake. However, to avoid dehydration and other health concerns, alcohol should be used in moderation.

In conclusion, hydration is a fundamental component of the Mediterranean diet, promoting the general health and energy of people in the region. Adherents of the Mediterranean diet improve their well-being and embrace a holistic approach to healthy living by prioritizing water and including herbal teas in their daily routines.

The Mediterranean Diet's Social And Lifestyle Aspects For Healthy Living

The Mediterranean diet covers a larger lifestyle approach that promotes social ties and a healthy way of life in addition to its focus on healthful meals. The Mediterranean diet's social and lifestyle features contribute greatly to the general well-being of people who follow this dietary pattern.

Meals are seen as a social occasion in Mediterranean cultures, bringing family and friends together. The act of eating together generates a sense of community and strong relationships.

This community eating method stresses the value of the social setting in boosting overall health and happiness, in addition to the nutritional quality of the meal.

The Mediterranean region's slower pace of life also contributes to the diet's effectiveness as a lifestyle choice. Slower eating allows people to enjoy their meals and identify sensations of fullness. This mindful eating technique develops a healthy connection with food and helps to prevent overeating. Furthermore, the emphasis on regular physical exercise, which is frequently incorporated into everyday activities, compliments the diet's overall lifestyle approach.

The Mediterranean way of life is defined by a strong connection to nature, with many people participating in outdoor activities and reaping the benefits of fresh air and sunlight. This link to the environment is consistent with the diet's emphasis on whole, unprocessed foods, emphasizing a comprehensive approach to health.

Another important part of the Mediterranean way of life is cultivating a good outlook. Simple pleasures, such as leisurely walks, time spent with loved ones, and appreciation of natural beauty, help to relieve stress and increase mental well-being.

To summarize, the Mediterranean diet is more than simply the meals on the plate; it is a way of life that includes social ties, mindful eating, and a well-balanced approach to health. Individuals who embrace the broader components of the Mediterranean way of life can benefit not just from the diet's physical health benefits, but also from a more fulfilled and joyous life.

Weight Control

The Mediterranean diet, which is well-known for its health advantages, is not just about enjoying wonderful food, but it also plays an important role in weight control. The cornerstone of this lifestyle is a diet rich in fruits, vegetables, whole grains, and olive oil while being modest in lean proteins and dairy. The emphasis on nutrient-dense, whole foods provides a satisfying and balanced eating style that aids with weight management.

The quantity of fiber in the Mediterranean diet is one of the primary elements leading to weight management. Whole grains, fruits, and vegetables are high in fiber, which promotes fullness and prevents overeating. Furthermore, the diet is low in processed foods and refined sugars, lowering the consumption of empty calories, which is commonly related to weight gain. The addition of heart-healthy fats from olive oil and almonds also aids in the maintenance of fullness.

Furthermore, the Mediterranean diet promotes conscious eating. Slowing down and enjoying meals enables for improved identification of hunger and fullness cues, which prevents mindless snacking. Regular physical exercise, a key component of the Mediterranean way of life, supplements the diet's advantages by promoting general well-being and assisting with weight management.

Precautions And Potential Health Risks

While the Mediterranean diet has been linked to several health advantages, it is essential to be aware of potential hazards and take the required measures.

One factor to consider is the drinking of red wine. While moderate red wine drinking is part of a healthy diet and has been related to heart health, excessive alcohol use is associated with health hazards such as liver disease and addiction. It is critical to follow prescribed recommendations and speak with healthcare specialists, especially if you have a pre-existing ailment or are taking medication.

Another thing to think about is the salt levels of certain Mediterranean foods. Traditional meals may use high-sodium foods like olives and feta cheese. Monitoring salt consumption is critical, especially for people who have hypertension or renal problems. Choosing low-sodium options and cooking at home gives you more control over your salt consumption.

Individuals with dietary limitations, such as gluten sensitivity or lactose intolerance, should exercise caution as well. While the Mediterranean diet is adaptable and diversified, certain modifications may be required to meet the needs of individuals. Consultation with a nutritionist or healthcare expert can assist in tailoring the diet to meet individual needs while maintaining general health advantages.

CHAPTER FOUR

A Mediterranean Diet For Every Stage Of Life

The Mediterranean diet's versatility makes it appropriate for all periods of life, from birth to old age. The emphasis on fresh, complete meals for children offers important nutrients for growth and development. Early exposure to a range of fruits, vegetables, and whole grains fosters good eating habits that can last a lifetime. As children grow, including lean foods like fish and chicken helps them get enough protein for muscular growth.

The Mediterranean diet promotes maintained energy levels and excellent health during youth and maturity. The quantity of antioxidants found in fruits and vegetables benefits skin health and may help to slow the aging process. The nutrient-rich components of the diet supply critical vitamins and minerals required for fetal growth in pregnant women.

The Mediterranean diet is still advantageous in old age. The emphasis on heart-healthy fats promotes cardiovascular health, which is critical for the elderly. Furthermore, the anti-inflammatory effects of the diet may benefit the management of aging-related illnesses such as arthritis. Adequate calcium and vitamin D consumption from dairy and seafood promotes bone health and reduces the risk of osteoporosis.

Including The Mediterranean Diet In Your Daily Life

Incorporating the Mediterranean diet into one's everyday life does not have to be difficult. Simple modifications in food selection and meal preparation may have a big influence on your overall health.

Begin by including more fruits and vegetables in your meals and substituting nuts or fresh fruit for packaged snacks. Switching to healthy grains like brown rice and quinoa increases fiber consumption.

Olive oil, a staple of the Mediterranean diet, can be substituted for other cooking oils. Drizzled over salads or used as a dip for whole-grain bread, it provides taste and beneficial fats. Choose lean foods such as fish and chicken, and minimize your consumption of red meat. Herbs and spices can be used in place of salt to enhance flavor without sacrificing health.

Meal planning and preparation are critical components of living the Mediterranean lifestyle. Set aside time each week for meal preparation, with an emphasis on different, nutrient-rich products. Experiment with traditional recipes or develop innovative dishes that adhere to the ideals of the diet.

Participating in communal meals with family and friends, another feature of Mediterranean culture, not only improves the eating experience but also builds social relationships, which contribute to general well-being.

Meal Plans For The Mediterranean Diet

Making Mediterranean-inspired dishes is both interesting and healthy. A Greek yogurt parfait with fresh berries, honey, and a sprinkling of almonds can be served for breakfast.

A tasty and nutritious lunch choice is a quinoa salad with cherry tomatoes, cucumber, olives, and feta cheese drizzled with olive oil. A delectable meal of grilled fish or chicken with roasted veggies and whole-grain couscous.

Snack on a handful of mixed nuts or dip carrot sticks or whole-grain crackers in hummus. For dessert, combine fresh fruit with a dollop of Greek yogurt. Experimenting with herbs and spices like oregano, basil, and garlic adds depth and flavor to foods without adding extra salt or bad fats.

Mediterranean Diet-Inspired Recipes

1. Salad with Chickpeas from the Mediterranean:

- Composition:

- 1 can be drained and rinsed chickpeas

- Halved cherry tomatoes

- Diced cucumber

- Finely sliced red onion

- Sliced Kalamata olives

- Crumbled Feta cheese

- chopped fresh parsley

- Extra virgin olive oil

- Fresh lemon juice

- Season to taste with salt and pepper.

- Directions:

• Toss together chickpeas, tomatoes, cucumber, red onion, olives, and feta in a large mixing basin.

• In a separate small mixing bowl, combine the olive oil, lemon juice, salt, and pepper.

• Pour the dressing over the salad and gently toss to incorporate.

• Before serving, sprinkle with fresh parsley.

2. Grilled Mediterranean Fish Tacos:

• Composition:

• Fillets of white fish (such as cod or tilapia)

• Tortillas made from whole grains

• Greek yogurt sauce (yogurt, lemon juice, garlic, and dill)

• Slaw (shredded cabbage, carrots, and red onion)

• Sliced cherry tomatoes

• Chopped fresh cilantro

- Extra virgin olive oil

- Seasonings: paprika, cumin, salt, and pepper

- Directions:

- Season the fillets of fish with olive oil, paprika, cumin, salt, and pepper.

- Grill the fish until it is well done.

- Warm the tortillas before filling them with grilled fish, cabbage slaw, cherry tomatoes, and a sprinkle of Greek yogurt sauce.

- Before serving, garnish with fresh cilantro.

Adopting the Mediterranean diet not only helps with weight loss but also improves general health and lifespan. Individuals may reap the multiple benefits of this rich and healthful lifestyle by making thoughtful choices, eating different and nutrient-dense foods, and enjoying meals with loved ones.

conclusion of the Mediterranean diet for a healthy lifestyle

Finally, adopting the Mediterranean diet appears to be a tasty path toward complete well-being. The combination of bright fruits and vegetables, heart-healthy olive oil, and lean proteins not only tantalizes the taste senses but also acts as a nutritional compass, guiding individuals to maximum health. Extensive study has demonstrated its ability to reduce the risk of chronic illnesses, build cardiovascular resilience, and promote lifespan.

The Mediterranean diet is more than simply a culinary option; it's a way of life that promotes moderation, balance, and the enjoyment of nutritious, nutrient-dense foods. Its concentration of omega-3 fatty acids, antioxidants, and fiber demonstrates its potential to nourish both the body and the mind.

This eating strategy emerges as a beacon of simplicity and sustainability as we traverse the difficulties of modern existence.

In a world where fad diets come and go, the Mediterranean diet has stood the test of time because it is based on centuries-old customs and the knowledge of generations. It's not just a means to a goal, but a long-term road to a better, more fulfilled life—one dish at a time.

THE END

www.ingramcontent.com/pod-product-compliance
Lightning Source LLC
Chambersburg PA
CBHW060821260726
48660CB00003B/1030